THE ULTIMATE OSTEOPOROSIS DIET COOKBOOK FOR SENIORS

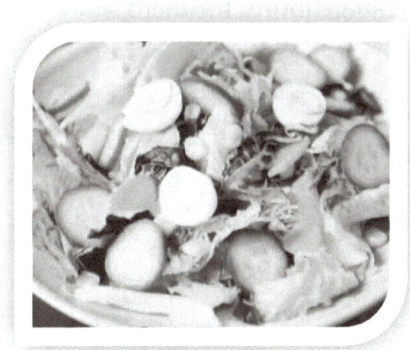

Delicious and Nutrient-Rich Recipes to naturally Combat Osteoporosis and Promote Bone Health for older people

Dr. Victoria Sterling

Text Copyright© 2023 by Dr. Victoria Sterling

All rights reserved worldwide No part of this publication may be republished in any form or by any means, including photocopying, scanning or otherwise without prior written permission to the copyright holder.

This book contains nonfictional content. The views expressed are those of the author and do not necessarily represent those of the publisher. In addition, the publisher declaims any responsibility for them.

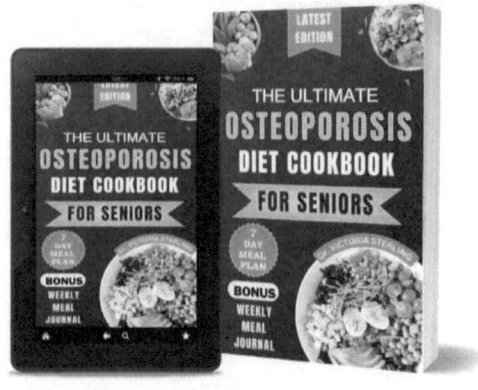

DEDICATION

To all those who have faced the silent struggles of osteoporosis,

This book is dedicated to you, the unsung heroes who have shown unwavering courage in the face of fragility, and resilience in the shadow of uncertainty. You are the inspiration behind these pages, and your strength has touched my heart in ways words cannot express.

To the countless individuals who have shared their stories, their fears, and their dreams with me, and to those who silently endure, this book is a tribute to your spirit. May the recipes within these pages not only nourish your bodies but also warm your souls with the promise of hope and healing.

In your journey, you've demonstrated that the human spirit can rise above adversity, that love and determination can conquer the most formidable challenges.

As you embrace this cookbook, may it be a companion on your path to stronger bones, better health, and a life filled with joy.

With profound gratitude and boundless hope,

Dr. Victoria Sterling

OTHER BOOKS BY THE AUTHOR

1. MEDITERRANEAN DIET COOKBOOK FOR CHRONIC KIDNEY DISEASE

CLICK HERE TO GET YOUR COPY!!!

2. MEDITERRANEAN TYPE-2 DIABETES DIET COOKBOOK FOR SENIORS

CLICK HERE TO GET YOUR COPY!!!

3. MEDITERRANEAN DASH DIET COOKBOOK FOR SENIORS

CLICK HERE TO GET YOUR COPY!!!

4. LOW-CARB ANTI-INFLAMMATORY DIET COOKBOOK FOR SENIORS

CLICK HERE TO GET YOUR COPY!!!

5. INSULIN RESISTANCE DIET COOKBOOK FOR WOMEN OVER 50

CLICK HERE TO GET YOUR COPY!!!

TABLE OF CONTENTS

INTRODUCTION 7

CHAPTER 1: 11

- ❖ Understanding Osteoporosis, the Silent Threat to Bone Health 11
- ❖ Types of Osteoporosis: 12
- ❖ Symptoms of Osteoporosis: 13
- ❖ Causes of Osteoporosis: 14
- ❖ Preventive Measures for Osteoporosis: 16

CHAPTER 2: 19

- ❖ Benefits of following Osteoporosis diet for seniors 19
- ❖ Foods to eat, limit, and avoid 23
- ❖ Complications of osteoporosis if the right diet isn't adopted 28

7-DAY MEAL PLAN 33

CHAPTER 3: 37

- ❖ **HEALING BREAKFAST RECIPES** 37
- ❖ **LUNCH RECIPES:** 49
- ❖ **DINNER RECIPES:** 59
- ❖ **JUICE AND SMOOTHIE RECIPES** 71

CONCLUSION 81
WEEKLY MEAL JOURNAL/ PLANNER

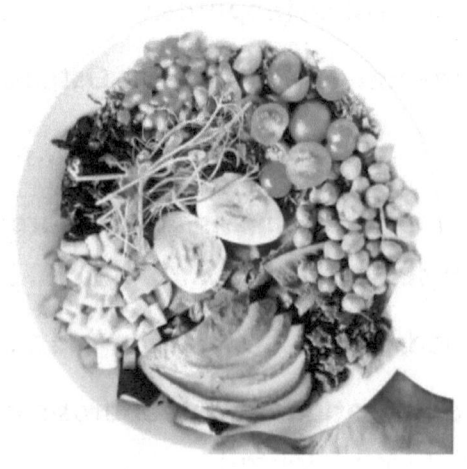

INTRODUCTION

Dear Reader,

I'm Dr. Victoria Sterling, a nutritionist with decades of experience, and I've seen the transformative power of food when it comes to our health. Today, I want to share a story with you, a story of hope, resilience, and the incredible ability of the human body to heal. It's a story of an old woman, a story that could be yours or that of a loved one.

In my years of practice, I met Mary, a graceful woman in her late 70s, who like many of us had her share of health challenges. But what weighed on her most was osteoporosis, a silent but devastating condition that had weakened her bones, leaving her fearful of the simplest of movements. Her once vibrant spirit was shackled by the fear of fractures and the pain that seemed never-ending.

Mary's struggle was a stark reminder that osteoporosis doesn't discriminate; it can affect anyone, particularly as we age. But her story doesn't end in despair. No, it's a testament to the power of the scientifically proven recipes you'll find in **"The Ultimate Osteoporosis Diet Cookbook for Seniors."**

I took Mary under my wing, determined to help her regain her strength and vitality. The journey was not without its challenges, but with the right foods, a dash of determination, and the love and care of her family, Mary began to transform. The nutrient-rich recipes in this cookbook became her allies in the fight against osteoporosis.

With time, Mary started to notice the changes. Her bones grew stronger, and the fear that had once imprisoned her began to fade. She could once again take long walks in the park, lift her grandchild without worry, and even dance at family gatherings.

The scientifically proven recipes in this cookbook provided Mary with a path to recovery that was not only effective but also delicious. You see, eating for bone health doesn't mean sacrificing taste. It means embracing a culinary journey filled with mouthwatering dishes designed to nourish your body and promote bone strength.

I'm sharing Mary's story with you because I want you to know that there is hope. Osteoporosis may be a formidable adversary, but you have the power to fight back. This cookbook is your ally, your guide to better bone health, and your key to a life of strength and independence.

Inside these pages, you'll discover recipes that will not only tantalize your taste buds but also provide your body with the essential nutrients it needs to combat osteoporosis. You'll learn about the foods that support bone health, how to create balanced meal plans, and valuable lifestyle tips to fortify your bones.

So, if you or a loved one is facing the challenge of osteoporosis, let this cookbook be your beacon of hope. With the right ingredients and a dash of determination, you can take the first step towards a life full of strength, joy, and the freedom to live on your own terms.

Welcome to **"The ·Ultimate Osteoporosis Diet Cookbook for Seniors."** Let's embark on this journey together, one delicious and nutrient-rich recipe at a time.

Yours in good health,

Dr. Victoria Sterling

CHAPTER 1:

Understanding Osteoporosis, the Silent Threat to Bone Health

Osteoporosis, often described as the "silent disease," is a common but often underdiagnosed condition that affects the bones. It is characterized by the weakening and thinning of bones, making them more prone to fractures and breaks. In this comprehensive exploration, we will delve into the various aspects of osteoporosis, including its types, causes, symptoms, and preventive measures, to empower you with the knowledge to protect your bone health and that of your loved ones.

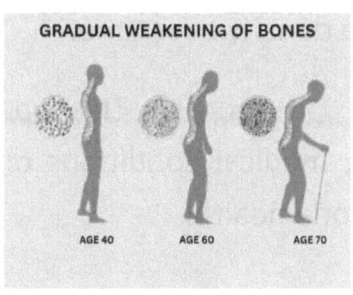

Types of Osteoporosis:

There are two primary types of osteoporosis:

1. **Primary Osteoporosis:** This type is more commonly associated with aging and hormonal changes. Within primary osteoporosis, there are two main categories:

   I. **Postmenopausal Osteoporosis:** Occurring predominantly in women after menopause, it is primarily due to the reduction of estrogen levels, which plays a key role in maintaining bone density.

   II. **Age-Related Osteoporosis:** Affecting both men and women, this type is linked to the natural aging process and the gradual loss of bone density over time.

2. **Secondary Osteoporosis:** This type is attributed to underlying medical conditions or medications that impact bone health.

Conditions such as hyperparathyroidism, malabsorption disorders, and long-term steroid use can lead to secondary osteoporosis.

Symptoms of Osteoporosis:

Osteoporosis often progresses silently, without obvious symptoms, until a fracture occurs. The most common fractures associated with osteoporosis are hip, spine, and wrist fractures. However, there are subtle signs that can signal the presence of osteoporosis, including:

1. Back Pain: Persistent back pain, often caused by fractures or the collapse of weakened vertebrae.

2. Loss of Height: Over time, osteoporosis can result in a gradual loss of height.

3. Stooped Posture: Known as "dowager's hump," this is a result of spine curvature due to fractures.

4. Bone Fractures: Fractures, especially in the hip, wrist, or spine, can occur more easily and with less force.

It's essential to remember that osteoporosis may remain asymptomatic for years, and early detection through bone density testing is crucial.

Causes of Osteoporosis:

Understanding the underlying causes of osteoporosis is crucial for both prevention and management. The primary factors contributing to the development of osteoporosis include:

1. Aging: As we age, our bones naturally lose density and become more susceptible to fractures.

2. Hormonal Changes: A significant factor in osteoporosis is hormonal fluctuations, particularly the reduction of estrogen in postmenopausal women. In men, a decrease in testosterone levels can also contribute to bone loss.

3. **Family History:** A family history of osteoporosis can increase one's risk.

4. **Dietary Choices:** Poor nutrition, low calcium intake, and vitamin D deficiency can all weaken bones.

5. **Lifestyle Factors:** Lack of physical activity, smoking, excessive alcohol consumption, and a sedentary lifestyle can exacerbate bone loss.

6. **Medical Conditions:** Certain medical conditions like hyperparathyroidism, rheumatoid arthritis, and gastrointestinal disorders can lead to secondary osteoporosis.

7. **Medications:** Long-term use of medications like corticosteroids, anticonvulsants, and some cancer treatments may weaken bones.

Preventive Measures for Osteoporosis:

The good news is that there are several preventive measures and lifestyle changes that can reduce the risk of osteoporosis:

1. **A Balanced Diet:** Ensure your diet is rich in calcium and vitamin D, essential for bone health. Dairy products, leafy greens, and fortified foods are excellent sources.

2. **Regular Exercise:** Weight-bearing exercises, such as walking, jogging, and strength training, can help build and maintain bone density.

3. **Lifestyle Choices:** Quit smoking and limit alcohol consumption, as both can contribute to bone loss.

4. **Bone Density Testing:** Regular bone density scans can help identify osteoporosis early, enabling timely intervention.

5. Medication: In some cases, healthcare providers may recommend medication to manage osteoporosis. These should be used in conjunction with lifestyle changes.

6. Fall Prevention: Take steps to reduce the risk of falls, such as ensuring well-lit spaces, using handrails, and removing tripping hazards at home.

7. Hormone Therapy: For postmenopausal women, hormone replacement therapy may be considered to help maintain bone density.

Osteoporosis is a complex condition that affects bone health, and understanding its types, causes, symptoms, and preventive measures is crucial in addressing this silent but significant threat. By adopting a bone-healthy lifestyle and seeking early diagnosis and treatment when needed, you can fortify your bones, reduce the risk of fractures, and enjoy a more active and independent life as you age. Remember, your bone health is an investment in your overall well-being.

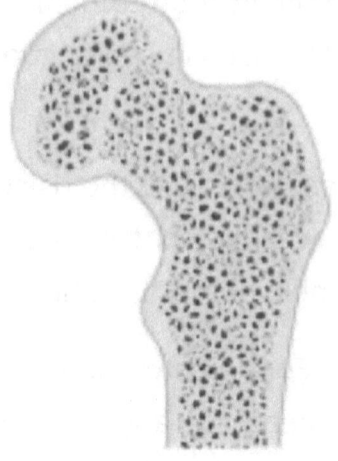

HEALTHY BONE

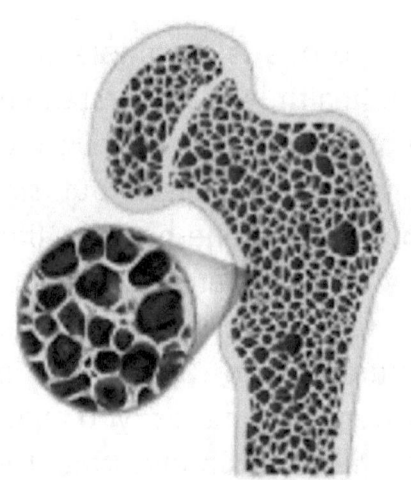

CHAPTER 2:

Benefits of following Osteoporosis diet for seniors

Following an osteoporosis diet for seniors can offer a range of core benefits that are essential for managing and preventing this condition. Here are the key advantages:

Improved Bone Health: An osteoporosis diet focuses on calcium and other essential nutrients like vitamin D, vitamin K, and magnesium, which are crucial for bone health. Consuming these nutrients helps to strengthen bones, reduce the risk of fractures, and slow down bone loss, ultimately enhancing bone density.

Reduced Fracture Risk: Strong bones are less prone to fractures. By maintaining optimal bone health through a well-balanced diet, seniors can significantly decrease their risk of experiencing debilitating fractures, especially common in osteoporosis.

Enhanced Muscle Function: A diet rich in protein, particularly from lean sources, supports muscle health. Strong muscles contribute to overall mobility and can help seniors maintain balance, reducing the risk of falls that may result in fractures.

Better Joint Health: Nutrient-dense foods, such as fruits and vegetables, contain antioxidants and anti-inflammatory compounds that can help manage joint pain and discomfort, which are often associated with osteoporosis.

Maintained Independence: Strong bones and muscles enable seniors to maintain their independence and continue with their daily activities without relying on assistance. This leads to a higher quality of life and greater self-sufficiency.

Enhanced Nutrient Absorption: An osteoporosis diet often includes foods that promote better nutrient absorption, such as those high in vitamin C. This facilitates the body's ability to utilize essential bone-strengthening nutrients effectively.

Heart Health: Many components of an osteoporosis diet, such as low-sodium choices and healthy fats, support cardiovascular health. Seniors can enjoy the dual benefit of better bone health and reduced risk of heart-related issues.

Weight Management: A balanced diet helps seniors maintain a healthy weight. Excess body weight can put unnecessary pressure on the bones and joints, while being underweight can increase the risk of fractures. An osteoporosis diet supports a healthy and stable weight.

Reduction in Medication Dependency: A well-managed diet can potentially reduce the need for medications to treat osteoporosis. This not only minimizes potential side effects but also enhances overall health and well-being.

Slower Progression of Osteoporosis: Following an osteoporosis diet, seniors can slow down the progression of the condition. This means they can better manage and control the symptoms and complications associated with osteoporosis.

Better Overall Nutrition: An osteoporosis diet encourages the consumption of nutrient-rich foods, which can lead to improved overall nutrition and overall well-being. It helps seniors get the essential vitamins and minerals they need for optimal health.

Lower Risk of Falls: Certain foods that support muscle strength and balance, such as those high in protein and calcium, can help seniors maintain their stability and reduce the risk of falling, a common trigger for fractures in older adults.

An osteoporosis diet for seniors offers a multi-faceted approach to managing and preventing the condition. It not only supports bone health but also promotes overall well-being, independence, and a better quality of life. By making dietary choices that prioritize essential nutrients, seniors can significantly enhance their physical health and reduce the risk of osteoporosis-related complications.

Foods to eat, limit, and avoid

Achieving and maintaining optimal bone and joint health is essential for overall well-being, and it becomes especially crucial when dealing with osteoporosis. A carefully crafted diet can be a powerful tool in managing this condition. In this guide, we'll explore the foods to eat, limit, and avoid promoting strong bones and joints.

Foods to Eat:

Dairy Products: Dairy items like milk, yogurt, and cheese are rich in calcium, a fundamental building block for bones. Opt for low-fat or non-fat versions to keep your saturated fat intake in check.

Leafy Greens: Vegetables like kale, broccoli, and collard greens are excellent sources of calcium and other essential nutrients like vitamin K, which aids in bone mineralization.

Fatty Fish: Salmon, mackerel, and sardines provide a healthy dose of vitamin D and omega-3 fatty acids, which support bone health.

Fortified Foods: Many foods, such as fortified cereals and orange juice, contain added calcium and vitamin D. These can be valuable additions to your diet.

Nuts and Seeds: Almonds, chia seeds, and sesame seeds offer calcium, magnesium, and other minerals that are crucial for bone health.

Lean Proteins: Incorporate lean sources of protein like poultry, tofu, and beans to maintain muscle and bone strength.

Whole Grains: Whole grains, such as brown rice and whole wheat bread, provide essential nutrients like magnesium, which plays a role in bone health.

Fruits: Fruits like oranges and berries contain vitamin C, which supports collagen production, vital for bone and joint health.

Low-Fat Dairy Alternatives: If you're lactose intolerant or prefer non-dairy options, choose fortified almond milk, soy milk, or other alternatives enriched with calcium and vitamin D.

Foods to Limit:

Red Meat: While lean cuts of red meat provide protein, they should be consumed in moderation. Excessive red meat intake can lead to an acidic environment in the body, potentially affecting bone health.

Salt: High-sodium diets can lead to calcium loss in the urine, which is detrimental to bone health. Reduce your salt intake by limiting processed and packaged foods.

Caffeine: Excessive caffeine consumption may contribute to calcium loss. Limit your intake of coffee, tea, and caffeinated sodas.

Soda and Sugary Beverages: These drinks often contain phosphoric acid, which can interfere with calcium absorption. Opt for healthier beverage choices like water or herbal teas.

Alcohol: Heavy alcohol consumption can weaken bones and increase the risk of fractures. If you choose to drink, do so in moderation.

Foods to Avoid:

Highly Processed Foods: Processed foods are often high in salt, sugar, and unhealthy fats, which can have a negative impact on overall health, including bone and joint health.

Trans Fats: Trans fats, found in many processed and fried foods, can lead to inflammation and may reduce bone density.

Excessive Sweets: High sugar intake can lead to inflammation and negatively affect the body's ability to absorb calcium.

Highly Acidic Foods: Foods that create an acidic environment in the body, such as excessive meat and certain grains, can potentially contribute to bone weakening.

Excessively Salty Snacks: Potato chips, pretzels, and other salty snacks can lead to high sodium intake, which may result in calcium loss.

In addition to your dietary choices, maintaining a healthy lifestyle is crucial for bone and joint health. Engage in weight-bearing exercises, such as walking or resistance training, to stimulate bone growth and maintain muscle strength. Adequate vitamin D intake, through sunlight exposure and supplements if necessary, is also vital, as it helps the body absorb calcium efficiently.

By making thoughtful food choices and embracing a holistic approach to bone and joint health, you can effectively manage osteoporosis and promote a higher quality of life. Remember, your diet is a key component in the journey to stronger bones and healthier joints.

Complications of osteoporosis if the right diet isn't adopted

Without the adoption of the right diet and appropriate management strategies, osteoporosis can lead to several serious complications. These complications can significantly impact a person's quality of life and overall health. Here are some of the most common complications associated with untreated or poorly managed osteoporosis:

Fractures: The primary and most immediate complication of osteoporosis is bone fractures. Weakened bones are much more susceptible to fractures, particularly in the hip, spine, and wrist. These fractures can result from even minor falls or everyday activities and can lead to pain, disability, and loss of independence.

Chronic Pain: Osteoporotic fractures, especially vertebral fractures, can cause chronic back pain.

This ongoing pain can significantly reduce a person's quality of life and make daily activities difficult.

Reduced Mobility: Fractures and chronic pain can lead to reduced mobility. This limitation in physical activity can result in muscle weakness and loss of balance, increasing the risk of falls and further fractures.

Kyphosis (Dowager's Hump): Multiple vertebral fractures can cause the spine to curve forward, resulting in a condition known as kyphosis or dowager's hump. This change in posture not only affects physical appearance but can also contribute to back pain and breathing difficulties.

Hospitalization: Fractures, particularly hip fractures, often require hospitalization and surgery. Hospital stays can be physically and emotionally challenging for individuals, especially seniors.

Surgical Complications: Surgical procedures to repair fractures come with their own set of risks and complications, such as infection, blood clots, and anesthesia-related issues.

Loss of Independence: Due to the pain, fractures, and mobility limitations, osteoporosis can lead to a loss of independence. Seniors may require assistance with daily activities, which can be emotionally distressing.

Psychological Impact: Osteoporosis-related complications can have a profound psychological impact, including depression, anxiety, and a diminished sense of well-being. Chronic pain, altered body image, and loss of independence contribute to these emotional challenges.

Decreased Quality of Life: All the complications mentioned above contribute to a decreased quality of life. Individuals may find it challenging to engage in social activities, exercise, or enjoy hobbies and interests they once cherished.

Increased Healthcare Costs: Managing complications of osteoporosis, including fractures, surgeries, and hospital stays, can lead to significant healthcare costs, placing a financial burden on individuals and healthcare systems.

Risk of Additional Fractures: Once an individual experiences an osteoporotic fracture, their risk of experiencing additional fractures increases. This is known as the "fracture cascade" and further compounds the health and financial burden.

It's important to note that osteoporosis is often preventable and manageable through lifestyle changes, including a bone-healthy diet, weight-bearing exercise, and appropriate medical interventions. Early detection and timely treatment can significantly reduce the risk of complications and help individuals maintain their bone health and overall well-being. Therefore, it is crucial for individuals at risk of osteoporosis to adopt preventive measures.

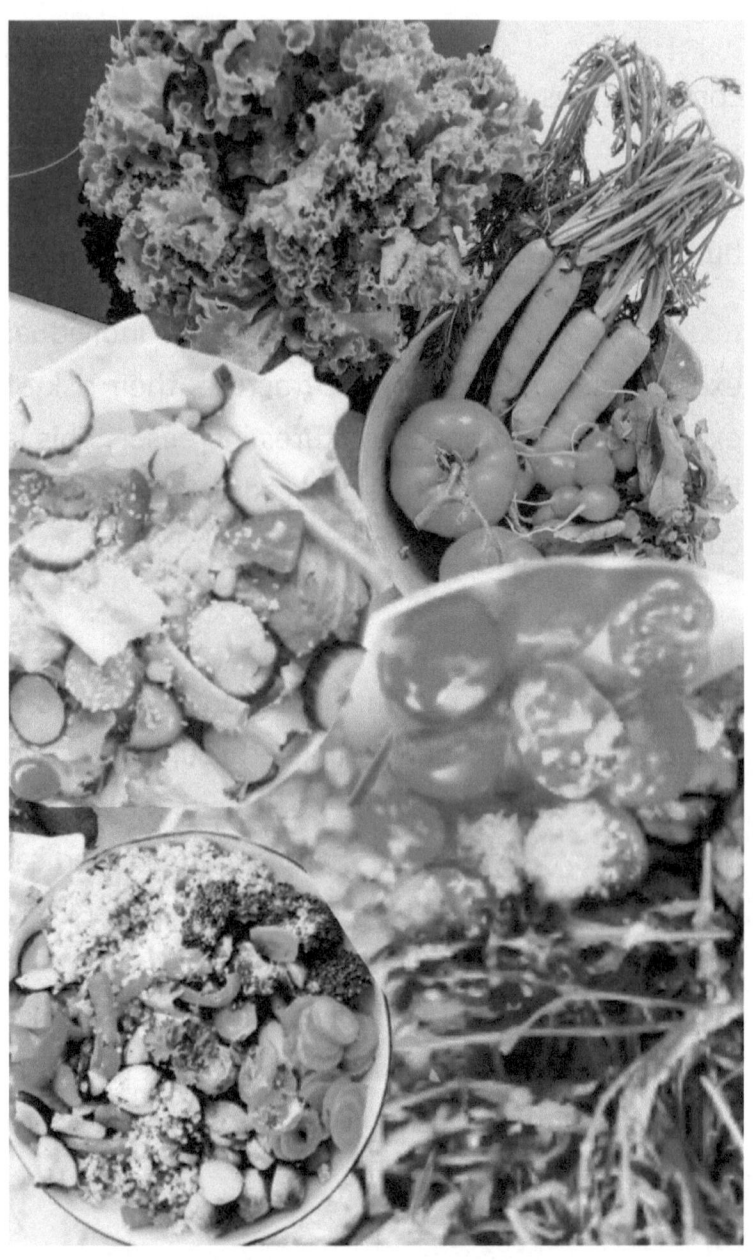

7-DAY MEAL PLAN

DAY 1:

BREAKFAST: **Creamy Greek Yogurt Parfait** (Page 37)

LUNCH: **Quinoa and Black Bean Bowl** (Page 50)

DINNER: **Baked Lemon Herb Tilapia** (Page 59)

DAY 2:

BREAKFAST: **Spinach and Feta Omelette** (Page 38)

LUNCH: **Grilled Chicken and Asparagus** (Page 52)

DINNER: Quinoa and Vegetable Stuffed Bell Peppers (Page 60)

DAY 3:

BREAKFAST: **Avocado and Tomato Toast**

(Page 40)

LUNCH: **Broccoli and Chickpea Stir-Fry**

(Page 54)

DINNER: **Vegetable and Quinoa Soup**

(Page 69)

DAY 4:

BREAKFAST: **Cottage Cheese and Berries Bowl** (Page 42)

LUNCH: **Tuna and White Bean Salad**

(Page 53)

DINNER: **Stuffed Acorn Squash**

(Page 64)

DAY 5:

BREAKFAST: **Banana and Almond Butter Smoothie**

(Page 41)

LUNCH: **Spinach and Salmon Salad**

(Page 49)

DINNER: **Turkey and Vegetable Stir-Fry**
(Page 63)

DAY 6:

BREAKFAST: **Blueberry and Almond Oatmeal**
(Page 44)

LUNCH: **Salmon and Vegetable Foil Pack**

(Page 57)

DINNER: **Chicken and Vegetable Skewers**

(Page 65)

DAY 7:

BREAKFAST: **Banana and Almond Butter Smoothie**

(Page 41)

LUNCH: **Sweet Potato and Kale Salad**

(Page 55)

DINNER: **Tofu and Vegetable Stir-Fry**

(Page 67)

CHAPTER 3:
HEALING BREAKFAST RECIPES

1. Creamy Greek Yogurt Parfait

Ingredients:

- 1 cup plain Greek yogurt
- 1/4 cup sliced strawberries
- 1 tablespoon chopped almonds
- 1 teaspoon honey (optional)
- 1/2 teaspoon chia seeds

Preparation:

1. In a bowl, layer the Greek yogurt, strawberries, and almonds.
2. Drizzle honey (if desired) and sprinkle chia seeds on top and Serve immediately.

Serving: 1 serving **Cooking Time:** 5 minutes

Nutritional Value: Calories: 260, Protein: 18g, Calcium: 250mg, Fiber: 4g

2. Spinach and Feta Omelette

Ingredients:

- 2 large eggs
- 1/4 cup fresh spinach, chopped
- 2 tablespoons crumbled feta cheese
- Salt and pepper to taste
- 1 teaspoon olive oil

Preparation:

1. In a mixing dish, whisk together the eggs and season with salt and pepper.
2. In a nonstick skillet, heat the olive oil over a moderate heat.
3. Add the spinach and Cook for about two minutes or until the spinach has wilted.
4. Pour the beaten eggs over the spinach and sprinkle feta cheese on top.
5. Cook until the omelette is set, then fold it in half and serve.

Serving: 1 serving   **Cooking Time:** 10 minutes

Nutritional Value: Calories: 270, Protein: 18g, Calcium: 140mg

3. Overnight Chia Seed Pudding

Ingredients:

- 3 tablespoons chia seeds
- 1 cup unsweetened almond milk
- 1/4 teaspoon vanilla extract
- 1/4 cup fresh berries
- 1 tablespoon chopped walnuts

Preparation:

1. In a jar, combine chia seeds, almond milk, and vanilla extract. Stir well.
2. Refrigerate the mixture for at least four hours or overnight.
3. Top with fresh berries and chopped walnuts before serving.

Serving: 1 serving

Nutritional Value: Calories: 220, Protein: 6g, Calcium: 350mg, Fiber: 10g

Cooking Time: 5 minutes (plus overnight refrigeration)

4. Avocado and Tomato Toast

Ingredients:

- 1 slice whole-grain bread
- 1/2 ripe avocado, mashed
- 1 small tomato, sliced
- Salt and pepper to taste

Preparation:

1. Toast the whole-grain bread.
2. Spread the mashed avocado on the toast.
3. Season with salt and pepper and serve with sliced tomatoes.

Serving: 1 serving   **Cooking Time:** 5 minutes

Nutritional Value: Calories: 230, Protein: 5g, Calcium: 40mg, Fiber: 6g

5. Banana and Almond Butter Smoothie

Ingredients:

- 1 ripe banana
- 1 tablespoon almond butter
- 1 cup unsweetened almond milk
- 1/2 teaspoon cinnamon
- 1 teaspoon honey (optional)

Preparation:

1. Blend all of the ingredients in a blender until smooth.
2. Add honey (if desired) for extra sweetness.

Serving: 1 serving

Nutritional Value: Calories: 280, Protein: 5g, Calcium: 200mg

Cooking Time: 5 minutes

6. Cottage Cheese and Berries Bowl

Ingredients:

- 1/2 cup low-fat cottage cheese
- 1/4 cup mixed berries (blueberries, strawberries, raspberries)
- 1 tablespoon chopped pecans
- 1/2 teaspoon honey (optional)

Preparation:

1. In a bowl, layer the cottage cheese and mixed berries.
2. Top with chopped pecans and drizzle with honey (if desired).

Serving: 1 serving   **Cooking Time:** 5 minutes

Nutritional Value: Calories: 250, Protein: 16g, Calcium: 200mg

7. Quinoa Breakfast Bowl

Ingredients:

- 1/2 cup cooked quinoa
- 1/4 cup sliced peaches
- 1 tablespoon pumpkin seeds
- 1 teaspoon honey (optional)

Preparation:

1. In a bowl, place the cooked quinoa.
2. Top with sliced peaches and pumpkin seeds.
3. Drizzle with honey (if desired).

Serving: 1 serving

Nutritional Value: Calories: 280, Protein: 7g, Calcium: 40mg, Fiber: 4g

Cooking Time: 15 minutes (for quinoa preparation)

8. Blueberry and Almond Oatmeal

Ingredients:

- 1/2 cup old-fashioned oats
- 1 cup unsweetened almond milk
- 1/4 cup fresh blueberries
- 1 tablespoon sliced almonds
- 1/2 teaspoon honey (optional)

Preparation:

1. Cook oats with almond milk according to package instructions.
2. Top with fresh blueberries, sliced almonds, and a drizzle of honey (if desired).

Serving: 1 serving   **Cooking Time:** 10 minutes

Nutritional Value: Calories: 280, Protein: 8g, Calcium: 200mg, Fiber: 6g

9. Sweet Potato and Spinach Breakfast Hash

Ingredients:

- 1 small sweet potato, diced
- 1 cup fresh spinach
- 1/4 cup diced red bell pepper
- 2 large eggs
- Salt and pepper to taste
- 1 teaspoon olive oil

Preparation:

1. In a pan, heat the olive oil over moderate heat.
2. Add diced sweet potato and cook until tender and slightly crispy, about 10 minutes.
3. Add in the red bell pepper and cook for two more minutes.

4. Add the fresh spinach, stir, and cook until it wilts.
5. Create two small wells in the hash and crack eggs into them.
6. Cook the eggs covered until they reach your desired liking.
7. Season with salt and pepper before serving.

Serving: 2 servings

Nutritional Value (per serving):

Calories: 280

Protein: 11g

Calcium: 80mg

Cooking Time: 20 minutes

10. Almond and Berry Quinoa Breakfast Bowl

Ingredients:

- 1/2 cup cooked quinoa
- 1/4 cup mixed berries (strawberries, blackberries, blueberries)
- 2 tablespoons sliced almonds
- 1/2 teaspoon honey (optional)

Preparation:

1. In a bowl, place the cooked quinoa.
2. Top with mixed berries and sliced almonds.
3. Drizzle with honey (if desired).

Serving: 1 serving

Nutritional Value:

- Calories: 290
- Protein: 8g
- Calcium: 60mg

- Fiber: 6g

Cooking Time: 15 minutes (for quinoa preparation)

These quick and easy breakfast recipes for seniors with osteoporosis are designed to provide essential nutrients for bone health while being diabetes- and heart healthy-friendly. They are delicious, convenient to prepare, and rich in the vitamins and minerals needed to support strong bones and overall well-being.

LUNCH RECIPES:

1. Spinach and Salmon Salad

Ingredients:

- 3 oz cooked salmon
- 2 cups fresh spinach
- 1/4 cup cherry tomatoes
- 1/4 cup cucumber slices
- 1 tablespoon olive oil and lemon juice
- Salt and pepper to taste

Preparation:

1. Flake the cooked salmon and set it aside.
2. In a large bowl, combine fresh spinach, cherry tomatoes, and cucumber slices.
3. Season with salt and pepper after drizzling with olive oil and lemon juice.
4. Top the salad with flaked salmon.

Serving: 1 serving   **Cooking Time:** 15 minutes

Nutritional Value: Calories: 250, Protein: 22g, Calcium: 200mg

2. Quinoa and Black Bean Bowl

Ingredients:

- 1/2 cup cooked quinoa
- 1/2 cup black beans, drained and rinsed
- 1/4 cup diced red bell pepper
- 1/4 cup corn kernels
- 1/4 cup diced avocado
- 1 tablespoon fresh lime juice
- 1/2 teaspoon cumin
- Salt and pepper to taste

Preparation:

1. In a bowl, combine cooked quinoa, black beans, red bell pepper, corn, and avocado.
2. Drizzle with fresh lime juice and sprinkle with cumin.
3. Season with salt and pepper and toss well.

Serving: 1 serving

Nutritional Value: Calories: 300, Protein: 11g, Calcium: 40mg

Cooking Time: 20 minutes (for quinoa preparation)

3. Lentil and Vegetable Soup

Ingredients:

- 1/2 cup dried green or brown lentils
- 1 cup mixed vegetables (carrots, celery, onions)
- 1 clove garlic, minced
- 4 cups low-sodium vegetable broth
- 1/2 teaspoon thyme
- Pinch of Salt and pepper to taste

Preparation:

1. Rinse and drain lentils.
2. In a pot, sauté mixed vegetables and garlic until soft.
3. Add lentils, vegetable broth, thyme, and season with salt and pepper.
4. Cook for twenty-five to thirty minutes or until the lentils are cooked.

Serving: 2 servings   **Cooking Time:** 45 minutes

Nutritional Value (per serving): Calories: 220, Protein: 10g, Calcium: 40mg

4. Grilled Chicken and Asparagus

Ingredients:

- 4 oz grilled chicken breast
- 1 cup asparagus spears
- 1/2 tablespoon olive oil
- 1/2 teaspoon garlic powder
- Lemon wedges for garnish
- Small Salt and pepper to taste

Preparation:

1. Season the chicken breast with garlic powder, salt, and pepper.
2. Grill the chicken until fully cooked.
3. In a separate pan, sauté asparagus in olive oil until tender.
4. Serve the grilled chicken with asparagus and garnish with lemon wedges.

Serving: 1 serving   **Cooking Time:** 20 minutes

Nutritional Value: Calories: 280, Protein: 30g, Calcium: 40mg

5. Tuna and White Bean Salad

Ingredients:

- 3 oz canned tuna in water, drained
- 1/2 cup canned white beans, drained and rinsed
- 1/4 cup diced red onion
- 1/4 cup chopped parsley
- 1 tablespoon olive oil and red wine vinegar
- Salt and pepper to taste

Preparation:

1. In a bowl, combine canned tuna, white beans, red onion, and parsley.
2. Drizzle with red wine vinegar and olive oil.
3. Season with salt and pepper, and mix to combine.

Serving: 1 serving   **Cooking Time:** 10 minutes

Nutritional Value: Calories: 270, Protein: 30g, Calcium: 100mg

6. Broccoli and Chickpea Stir-Fry

Ingredients:

- 1 cup broccoli florets
- 1/2 cup canned chickpeas, drained and rinsed
- 1/4 cup sliced red bell pepper
- 1/4 cup sliced mushrooms
- 2 tablespoons low-sodium soy sauce
- 1 teaspoon sesame oil
- 1/2 teaspoon ginger

Preparation:

1. In a pan, stir-fry broccoli, chickpeas, red bell pepper, and mushrooms with sesame oil and ginger until tender.
2. Drizzle with low-sodium soy sauce and stir-fry for an additional minute.

Serving: 1 serving   **Cooking Time:** 15 minutes

Nutritional Value: Calories: 280, Protein: 12g, Calcium: 50mg

7. Sweet Potato and Kale Salad

Ingredients:

- 1 cup roasted sweet potato cubes
- 2 cups chopped kale
- 1/4 cup dried cranberries
- 1/4 cup chopped pecans
- 1 tablespoon balsamic vinaigrette
- Salt and pepper to taste

Preparation:

1. In a bowl, combine roasted sweet potato, chopped kale, dried cranberries, and pecans.
2. Season with salt and pepper and drizzle with balsamic vinaigrette.

Serving: 1 serving

Nutritional Value: Calories: 310, Protein: 5g, Calcium: 80mg

Cooking Time: 30 minutes (for sweet potato roasting)

8. Egg and Vegetable Wrap

Ingredients:

- 2 large eggs, 1 whole-grain tortilla
- 1/4 cup diced bell peppers
- 1/4 cup diced onions
- 1/4 cup diced tomatoes
- 1/4 cup chopped spinach
- 1/4 cup low-fat cheese (optional)
- Salt and pepper to taste

Preparation:

1. In a mixing dish, whisk together the eggs and season with salt and pepper.
2. In a pan, sauté bell peppers, onions, and tomatoes until soft.
3. Add the beaten eggs and cook until set.
4. Lay the egg mixture on the tortilla, top with chopped spinach and cheese (if desired), and wrap.

Serving: 1 serving   **Cooking Time:** 15 minutes

Nutritional Value: Calories: 330, Protein: 17g, Calcium: 150mg

9. Salmon and Vegetable Foil Pack

Ingredients:

- 4 oz salmon fillet
- 1/2 cup broccoli florets
- 1/2 cup carrot slices
- 1/4 cup red onion slices
- 1/2 tablespoon olive oil
- 1/2 teaspoon lemon zest
- Salt and pepper to taste

Preparation:

1. Preheat the oven to 375°F (190°C).
2. Place salmon, broccoli, carrots, and red onions on a large piece of aluminum foil.
3. Drizzle with olive oil and lemon zest, and season with salt and pepper.
4. Seal the foil into a packet and bake for 20-25 minutes, until the salmon is cooked through.

Serving: 1 serving   **Cooking Time:** 25 minutes

Nutritional Value: Calories: 320, Protein: 25g, Calcium: 150mg

10. Mediterranean Hummus Wrap

Ingredients:

- 1 whole-grain tortilla
- 2 tablespoons hummus
- 2 slices roasted red pepper
- 1/4 cup cucumber slices
- 1/4 cup mixed greens
- 1/4 cup crumbled feta cheese (optional)

Preparation:

1. Spread hummus on the whole-grain tortilla.
2. Layer with roasted red pepper, cucumber slices, mixed greens, and crumbled feta cheese (if desired).
3. Roll up the tortilla into a wrap.

Serving: 1 serving   **Cooking Time:** 10 minutes

Nutritional Value: Calories: 280, Protein: 8g, Calcium: 100mg

DINNER RECIPES:

1. Baked Lemon Herb Tilapia

Ingredients:

- 4 oz tilapia fillet, 1 lemon, thinly sliced
- 1 teaspoon olive oil
- 1/2 teaspoon dried herbs (e.g., thyme, rosemary, oregano)
- Salt and pepper to taste

Preparation:

1. Preheat the oven to 375°F (190°C).
2. Place the tilapia fillet on a baking sheet.
3. Drizzle with olive oil, sprinkle with dried herbs, and season with salt and pepper.
4. Top with lemon slices.
5. Bake the fish for fifteen to twenty minutes, or until it is flaky.

Serving: 1 serving   **Cooking Time:** 20 minutes

Nutritional Value: Calories: 220, Protein: 25g, Calcium: 40mg

2. Quinoa and Vegetable Stuffed Bell Peppers

Ingredients:

- 2 large bell peppers
- 1/2 cup cooked quinoa
- 1/4 cup black beans, drained and rinsed
- 1/4 cup diced tomatoes
- 1/4 cup diced zucchini
- 1/4 cup low-sodium vegetable broth
- 1/2 teaspoon cumin
- Salt and pepper to taste

Preparation:

1. Preheat the oven to 375°F (190°C).
2. Remove the seeds and cut off the bell peppers' tops.
3. In a bowl, combine cooked quinoa, black beans, diced tomatoes, diced zucchini, vegetable broth, cumin, salt, and pepper.
4. Place the quinoa mixture inside the bell peppers.

5. The filled peppers should be put on a baking tray and covered with foil.
6. Bake the peppers for thirty to thirty-five minutes, or until they are soft.

Serving: 2 servings

Nutritional Value (per serving):

- Calories: 250
- Protein: 8g
- Calcium: 60mg
- Cooking Time: 45 minutes

3. Lentil and Spinach Curry

Ingredients:

- 1/2 cup dried green lentils
- 1 cup fresh spinach
- 1/2 cup diced tomatoes
- 1/4 cup diced onions
- 1 clove garlic, minced
- 1 teaspoon curry powder
- Salt and pepper to taste

Preparation:

1. Rinse and drain lentils.
2. Add the garlic and onions to a saucepan and cook until tender.
3. Add diced tomatoes, curry powder, salt, and pepper.
4. Stir in lentils and simmer for 20-25 minutes until lentils are tender.
5. Add fresh spinach and cook until wilted.

Serving: 2 servings   **Cooking Time:** 45 minutes

Nutritional Value (per serving): Calories: 280, Protein: 15g, Calcium: 40mg

4. Turkey and Vegetable Stir-Fry

Ingredients:

- 4 oz ground turkey
- 1 cup mixed vegetables (e.g., broccoli, bell peppers, snap peas)
- 1/4 cup sliced mushrooms
- 1/4 cup low-sodium teriyaki sauce
- 1 teaspoon sesame oil, 1/2 teaspoon ginger

Preparation:

1. Cook the ground turkey in a pan until browned.
2. Add mixed vegetables and mushrooms, stir-fry until tender.
3. Drizzle with teriyaki sauce and sesame oil.
4. Sprinkle with ginger and cook for an additional minute.

Serving: 1 serving   **Cooking Time:** 15 minutes

Nutritional Value: Calories: 290, Protein: 20g, Calcium: 60mg

5. Stuffed Acorn Squash

Ingredients:

- 1 acorn squash, halved and seeds removed
- 1/2 cup cooked quinoa
- 1/4 cup chopped walnuts
- 1/4 cup dried cranberries
- 1/2 teaspoon cinnamon
- Salt and pepper to taste

Preparation:

1. Preheat the oven to 375°F (190°C).
2. The Acorn Squash halves should be put on a baking pan.
3. In a bowl, combine cooked quinoa, chopped walnuts, dried cranberries, cinnamon, salt, and pepper.
4. Stuff the acorn squash halves with the quinoa mixture.
5. Bake the squash for thirty to thirty-five minutes, or until it is soft.

Serving: 2 servings   **Cooking Time:** 45 minutes

Nutritional Value (per serving): Calories: 270, Protein: 6g, Calcium: 80mg

6. Chicken and Vegetable Skewers

Ingredients:

- 4 oz chicken breast, cut into chunks
- 1 cup bell pepper chunks
- 1/2 cup red onion chunks
- 1/2 cup zucchini chunks
- 1 tablespoon olive oil
- 1/2 teaspoon garlic powder
- Salt and pepper to taste

Preparation:

1. Preheat the grill or use a grill pan.
2. Thread chicken and vegetables onto skewers.
3. Add a drizzle of olive oil and season with salt, pepper, and garlic powder.
4. Grill for 10-15 minutes, or until chicken is cooked through and vegetables are tender.

Serving: 2 servings   **Cooking Time:** 15 minutes

Nutritional Value (per serving): Calories: 260, Protein: 30g, Calcium: 40mg

7. Chickpea and Spinach Curry

Ingredients:

- 1/2 cup canned chickpeas, drained and rinsed
- 1 cup fresh spinach
- 1/4 cup diced tomatoes
- 1/4 cup diced onions
- 1 clove garlic, minced
- 1 teaspoon curry powder
- Salt and pepper to taste

Preparation:

1. Add the garlic and onions to a saucepan and cook until tender.
2. Add diced tomatoes, curry powder, salt, and pepper.
3. Stir in chickpeas and simmer for 10-15 minutes.
4. Add fresh spinach and cook until wilted.

Serving: 2 servings   **Cooking Time:** 30 minutes

Nutritional Value (per serving): Calories: 240, Protein: 8g, Calcium: 80mg

8. Tofu and Vegetable Stir-Fry

Ingredients:

- 4 oz firm tofu, cubed
- 1 cup mixed vegetables (e.g., broccoli, carrots, snap peas)
- 1/4 cup sliced mushrooms
- 2 tablespoons low-sodium soy sauce
- 1 teaspoon sesame oil, 1/2 teaspoon ginger

Preparation:

1. In a pan, stir-fry tofu until golden.
2. Add mixed vegetables and mushrooms, stir-fry until tender.
3. Drizzle with sesame oil and low-sodium soy sauce.
4. Sprinkle with ginger and cook for an additional minute.

Serving: 1 serving   **Cooking Time:** 15 minutes

Nutritional Value: Calories: 280, Protein: 18g, Calcium: 60mg

9. Salmon and Broccoli Foil Pack

Ingredients:

- 4 oz salmon fillet
- 1 cup broccoli florets
- 1/2 cup sliced red bell pepper
- 1/2 tablespoon olive oil
- 1/2 teaspoon lemon zest
- Salt and pepper to taste

Preparation:

1. Preheat the oven to 375°F (190°C).
2. Place salmon, broccoli, and red bell pepper on a large piece of aluminum foil.
3. Drizzle with olive oil, lemon zest, and season with salt and pepper.
4. Seal the foil into a packet and bake for 20-25 minutes, until the salmon is cooked through.

Serving: 1 serving   **Cooking Time:** 25 minutes

Nutritional Value: Calories: 290, Protein: 25g, Calcium: 60mg

10. Vegetable and Quinoa Soup

Ingredients:

- 1/2 cup cooked quinoa
- 1 cup mixed vegetables (e.g., carrots, celery, green beans)
- 1/4 cup diced onions
- 1 clove garlic, minced
- 4 cups low-sodium vegetable broth
- 1/2 teaspoon thyme
- Salt and pepper to taste

Preparation:

1. Add the garlic and onions to a saucepan and cook until tender.
2. Add mixed vegetables, quinoa, vegetable broth, thyme, salt, and pepper.
3. Simmer for 20-25 minutes until vegetables are tender.

Serving: 2 servings   **Cooking Time:** 45 minutes

Nutritional Value (per serving): Calories: 230, Protein: 6g, Calcium: 40mg

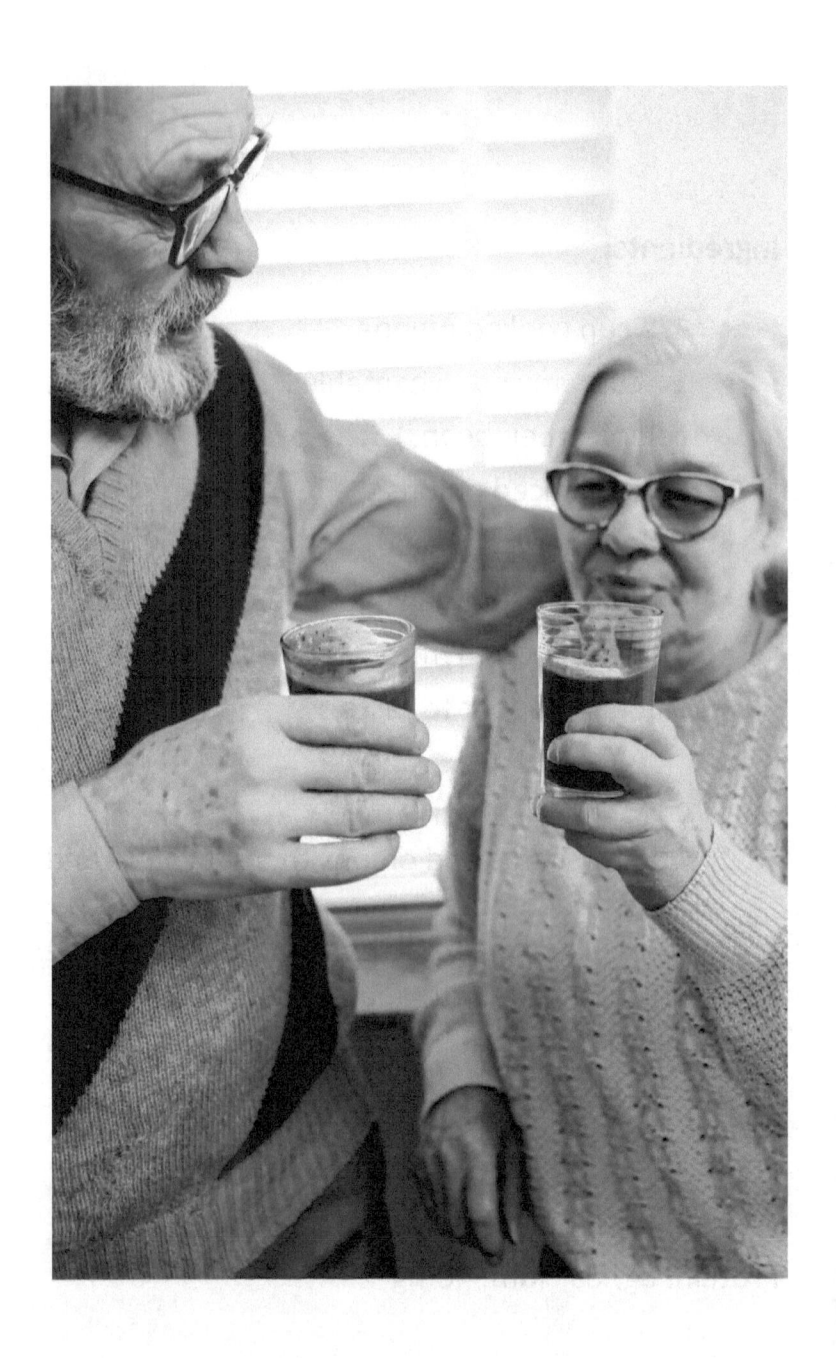

JUICE AND SMOOTHIE RECIPES

1. Berry Bliss Smoothie

Ingredients:

- 1/2 cup mixed berries (blueberries, strawberries, raspberries)
- 1/2 cup low-fat Greek yogurt
- 1/2 cup almond milk (unsweetened)
- 1 tablespoon chia seeds
- 1 teaspoon honey (optional)

Preparation:

1. Blend mixed berries, Greek yogurt, almond milk, and chia seeds until smooth.
2. Add honey for sweetness if desired.

Serving: 1 serving

Nutritional Value: Calories: 180, Protein: 12g, Calcium: 250mg

2. Green Goddess Smoothie

Ingredients:

- 1 cup fresh spinach
- 1/2 cup pineapple chunks
- 1/2 banana
- 1/2 cup low-fat Greek yogurt
- 1/2 cup water

Preparation:

1. Blend fresh spinach, pineapple chunks, banana, low-fat Greek yogurt, and water until smooth.

Serving: 1 serving

Nutritional Value:

- Calories: 180
- Protein: 10g
- Calcium: 220mg

3. Citrus Delight Juice

Ingredients:

- 1 orange, peeled
- 1/2 grapefruit, peeled
- 1 lemon, peeled
- 1/2 lime, peeled

Preparation:

1. Juice the orange, grapefruit, lemon, and lime.
2. Stir well and serve over ice.

Serving: 1 serving

Nutritional Value:

- Calories: 100
- Protein: 2g
- Calcium: 60mg

4. Tropical Twist Smoothie

Ingredients:

- 1/2 cup pineapple chunks
- 1/2 banana
- 1/2 cup low-fat coconut milk
- 1/2 cup low-fat Greek yogurt
- 1/2 cup water

Preparation:

1. Blend pineapple chunks, banana, low-fat coconut milk, low-fat Greek yogurt, and water until smooth.

Serving: 1 serving

Nutritional Value:

- Calories: 200
- Protein: 8g
- Calcium: 180mg

5. Kale and Kiwi Smoothie

Ingredients:

- 1 cup fresh kale
- 2 kiwis, peeled and sliced
- 1/2 cup low-fat Greek yogurt
- 1/2 cup water

Preparation:

1. Blend fresh kale, kiwis, low-fat Greek yogurt, and water until smooth.

Serving: 1 serving

Nutritional Value:

- Calories: 190
- Protein: 9g
- Calcium: 200mg

6. Berry Banana Boost Smoothie

Ingredients:

- 1/2 cup mixed berries (blueberries, strawberries, raspberries)
- 1/2 banana
- 1/2 cup low-fat Greek yogurt
- 1/2 cup almond milk (unsweetened)
- 1 tablespoon flaxseeds

Preparation:

1. Blend mixed berries, banana, low-fat Greek yogurt, almond milk, and flaxseeds until smooth.

Serving: 1 serving

Nutritional Value: Calories: 190, Protein: 12g

Calcium: 230mg

7. Carrot and Ginger Elixir

Ingredients:

- 2 large carrots
- 1-inch piece of fresh ginger
- 1 apple, cored and sliced
- 1/2 lemon, peeled

Preparation:

1. Juice the carrots, ginger, apple, and lemon.
2. Stir well and serve over ice.

Serving: 1 serving

Nutritional Value:

- Calories: 120
- Protein: 2g
- Calcium: 60mg

8. Creamy Avocado Green Smoothie

Ingredients:

- 1/2 avocado
- 1 cup fresh spinach
- 1/2 banana
- 1/2 cup almond milk (unsweetened)
- 1/2 cup low-fat Greek yogurt
- 1 teaspoon honey (optional)

Preparation:

1. Blend avocado, fresh spinach, banana, almond milk, low-fat Greek yogurt, and honey (if desired) until smooth.

Serving: 1 serving

Nutritional Value:

- Calories: 220
- Protein: 10g
- Calcium: 240mg

9. Apple Cinnamon Spice Smoothie

Ingredients:

- 1 apple, cored and sliced
- 1/2 teaspoon ground cinnamon
- 1/2 cup low-fat Greek yogurt
- 1/2 cup almond milk (unsweetened)
- 1 tablespoon oats

Preparation:

1. Blend apple slices, ground cinnamon, low-fat Greek yogurt, almond milk, and oats until smooth.

Serving: 1 serving

Nutritional Value:

- Calories: 200
- Protein: 8g
- Calcium: 220mg

10. Pomegranate Berry Blast Smoothie

Ingredients:

- 1/2 cup pomegranate seeds
- 1/2 cup mixed berries (blueberries, strawberries, raspberries)
- 1/2 cup low-fat Greek yogurt
- 1/2 cup water

Preparation:

1. Blend pomegranate seeds, mixed berries, low-fat Greek yogurt, and water until smooth.

Serving: 1 serving

These juice and smoothie recipes for seniors are not only delectable but also packed with nutrients to support bone health and overall well-being. Incorporate these into your daily routine to harness the benefits of scientifically proven ingredients for managing osteoporosis. Enjoy these refreshing beverages as a delightful addition to your osteoporosis diet.

CONCLUSION

"The Ultimate Osteoporosis Diet Cookbook for Seniors" is a labor of love, meticulously crafted to empower you with the knowledge and recipes you need to take charge of your bone health and overall well-being. Osteoporosis may seem like an intimidating foe, but with the right tools and guidance, you can stand strong in the face of this condition.

Throughout this cookbook, we've explored the nature of osteoporosis, its causes, symptoms, and preventive measures. We've delved into the importance of a diet that's not only delicious but scientifically proven to manage osteoporosis. You've discovered a treasure trove of nutrient-rich recipes, from breakfast to dinner, Juice to smoothies, all carefully designed to support your bone health while aligning with diabetes- and heart disease-friendly, kidney-friendly diets.

This isn't just about following a diet; it's about embracing a lifestyle that empowers you to live life to the fullest. It's about savoring every bite of these delicious recipes, knowing that each one is a step toward stronger bones, greater vitality, and a more fulfilling future.

Imagine yourself feeling more agile, standing tall, and embracing life's adventures with confidence. Picture yourself relishing the delicious flavors of these recipes while knowing that every bite is nurturing your body and helping you combat osteoporosis.

You hold the key to your own well-being, and this cookbook is your trusted guide. Embrace it, experiment with the recipes, and make them a part of your daily routine. Your bones will thank you, and your future self will be grateful for the choice you made today.

So, my dear reader, don't wait. Start this journey to better bone health and a more vibrant life.

The power is in your hands, and I believe in your ability to thrive. You are strong, and your journey towards a healthier, more fulfilling life begins with every recipe you create from these pages.

Embrace it, and let the transformation begin.

MY WEEKLY MEAL PLANNER

DATE: _____

DAYS	BREAKFAST	LUNCH	DINNER
MON			
TUE			
WED			
THU			
FRI			
SAT			
SUN			

SHOPPING LIST

- _____
- _____
- _____
- _____
- _____

NOTES

MY WEEKLY MEAL PLANNER

DATE: _____

DAYS	BREAKFAST	LUNCH	DINNER
MON			
TUE			
WED			
THU			
FRI			
SAT			
SUN			

SHOPPING LIST

- _____
- _____
- _____
- _____
- _____

NOTES

MY WEEKLY MEAL PLANNER

DATE: _____

DAYS	BREAKFAST	LUNCH	DINNER
MON			
TUE			
WED			
THU			
FRI			
SAT			
SUN			

SHOPPING LIST

- _____
- _____
- _____
- _____
- _____

NOTES

MY WEEKLY MEAL PLANNER

DATE: _____

DAYS	BREAKFAST	LUNCH	DINNER
MON			
TUE			
WED			
THU			
FRI			
SAT			
SUN			

SHOPPING LIST

- _____
- _____
- _____
- _____
- _____

NOTES

MY WEEKLY MEAL PLANNER

DATE:

DAYS	BREAKFAST	LUNCH	DINNER
MON			
TUE			
WED			
THU			
FRI			
SAT			
SUN			

SHOPPING LIST

-
-
-
-

NOTES

MY WEEKLY MEAL PLANNER

DATE: _____

DAYS	BREAKFAST	LUNCH	DINNER
MON			
TUE			
WED			
THU			
FRI			
SAT			
SUN			

SHOPPING LIST

- _____
- _____
- _____
- _____
- _____

NOTES

MY WEEKLY MEAL PLANNER

DATE: _____

DAYS	BREAKFAST	LUNCH	DINNER
MON			
TUE			
WED			
THU			
FRI			
SAT			
SUN			

SHOPPING LIST

- _____
- _____
- _____
- _____
- _____

NOTES

MY WEEKLY MEAL PLANNER

DATE: _____

DAYS	BREAKFAST	LUNCH	DINNER
MON			
TUE			
WED			
THU			
FRI			
SAT			
SUN			

SHOPPING LIST

- _____
- _____
- _____
- _____
- _____

NOTES

MY WEEKLY MEAL PLANNER

DATE:

DAYS	BREAKFAST	LUNCH	DINNER
MON			
TUE			
WED			
THU			
FRI			
SAT			
SUN			

SHOPPING LIST

- _____
- _____
- _____
- _____

NOTES

MY WEEKLY MEAL PLANNER

DATE: _____

DAYS	BREAKFAST	LUNCH	DINNER
MON			
TUE			
WED			
THU			
FRI			
SAT			
SUN			

SHOPPING LIST

- _____
- _____
- _____
- _____
- _____

NOTES

MY WEEKLY MEAL PLANNER

DATE: _____

DAYS	BREAKFAST	LUNCH	DINNER
MON			
TUE			
WED			
THU			
FRI			
SAT			
SUN			

SHOPPING LIST

- _____
- _____
- _____
- _____
- _____

NOTES

MY WEEKLY MEAL PLANNER

DATE:

DAYS	BREAKFAST	LUNCH	DINNER
MON			
TUE			
WED			
THU			
FRI			
SAT			
SUN			

SHOPPING LIST

-
-
-
-
-

NOTES

MY WEEKLY MEAL PLANNER

DATE:

DAYS	BREAKFAST	LUNCH	DINNER
MON			
TUE			
WED			
THU			
FRI			
SAT			
SUN			

SHOPPING LIST

-
-
-
-

NOTES

MY WEEKLY MEAL PLANNER

DATE:

DAYS	BREAKFAST	LUNCH	DINNER
MON			
TUE			
WED			
THU			
FRI			
SAT			
SUN			

SHOPPING LIST

-
-
-
-
-

NOTES

MY WEEKLY MEAL PLANNER

DATE: _____

DAYS	BREAKFAST	LUNCH	DINNER
MON			
TUE			
WED			
THU			
FRI			
SAT			
SUN			

SHOPPING LIST

- _____
- _____
- _____
- _____
- _____

NOTES

MY WEEKLY MEAL PLANNER

DATE: _____

DAYS	BREAKFAST	LUNCH	DINNER
MON			
TUE			
WED			
THU			
FRI			
SAT			
SUN			

SHOPPING LIST

- _____
- _____
- _____
- _____
- _____

NOTES

MY WEEKLY MEAL PLANNER

DATE:

DAYS	BREAKFAST	LUNCH	DINNER
MON			
TUE			
WED			
THU			
FRI			
SAT			
SUN			

SHOPPING LIST

-
-
-
-

NOTES

Made in United States
Troutdale, OR
02/21/2024